Dr. Anil Malleshi Betigeri

Quality design
in
Anatomical
Path**olog**y

Title:	*Quality design in Anatomical Pathology*
	by *Dr. Anil Malleshi Betigeri*
ISBN-13:	978-1466470262
ISBN-10:	1466470267
Cover design and Layout:	Elizabeth Log
	elizbeth.log@hotmail.com
Publisher:	**Internet Medical Publishing**
	info@imedpub.com
	http://imedpub.com/
First edition:	**2011**

Dr. **Anil** Malleshi Betigeri

Quality design in Anatomical Pathology

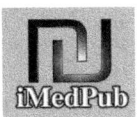
iMedPub

Index

Butterfly effect
and quality

Butterfly effect
and quality

The butterfly effect, as defined in the Chaos theory is an interesting phenomenon characterized by the sensitive dependence on initial conditions, wherein a small initial change at a place in a non-linear system can result in massive differences to a later state. The classical example quoted is that of a butterfly flapping its wings and causing a hurricane. Edward Lorenz popularized this term in weather forecasting which had already been described in the literature in a particular case of the three-body problem by Henri Poincaré in 1890. (Some Historical Notes: History of Chaos Theory) He observed that a very minute changes in one of the variables (instead of entering a value as 0.506127, he chose 0.506) in a computer model for weather forecasting affected the whole system tremendously.

The butterfly effect has been well appreciated in weather forecasting. However, in medical science, its potential has remained largely unexplored. Pathologists familiar with the intricacies of quality process in anatomical pathology would certainly relate to this effect when it comes to precision and accuracy in their pathology reports.

This is all the more important since the biological system follows non-linear dynamics where the output may not be directly proportional to its input. To a certain extent though, the biological system also follows laws of physics and biologists believe that exact modelling of a cell or biological system is possible. The fractal model of cancer growth has been generated by various scientists [2]. Different cell models and biological systems have been generated by researchers based on enormous data and findings [3, 4].

The prediction of different physiological and pathological phenomena is possible using non-linear dynamics such as deterministic chaos though it must not be forgotten that chaotic systems are highly responsive to initial conditions and a negligible input or apparently minor variation in the measurement of the basal state of system may produce an unexpected output; the butterfly effect.

For instance, the nucleus is the centre of all genetic material and this is where the initial genetic or epigenetic changes may occur in the event of a non-lethal cellular injury [5]. As has been documented during the process of carcinogenesis, mutations may happen within the nuclei of a single or a handful of cells. These may appear to be minor changes of negligible significance in the overall context of the organ system. However, the resulting cascade of functional derangements could lead to serious consequences and with the progression of time, affect the system tremendously culminating in the ultimate collapse of the entire system in a manner reminiscent of the butterfly effect [6].

In practicing anatomic pathology, the pathology report is a reflection of the pathologist's competence, based on the precision and accuracy involved in finalizing it. While there can be no doubt that the data provided by practitioners of anatomic pathology is highly relevant and valuable to the practice of evidence based medicine in the clinical arena one would do well to keep in mind that the knowledge base in this speciality is predominantly observational; which can create a butterfly effect in clinical outcome. Moreover, from a phenotypic-clinical framework of diagnosis, we are shifting into a phenotypic-molecular-clinical dimension [7].

Conclusions

The majority of studies on the quality of oncologic pathology diagnoses have focused on patient safety and have documented a variety of causes of errors that occur in the clinical and anatomic pathology department testing phases. Clinical practitioners play an essential role in error reduction through several avenues such as effective test ordering, providing accurate and pertinent clinical information, procuring high-quality specimens, providing timely follow-up on test results, effectively communicating on potentially discrepant diagnoses, and advocating second opinions on the pathology diagnosis in specific situations.

This is indeed the right time to consider a re-look into the functioning of our anatomic pathology departments, especially in light of litigation threats looming large over today's medical practice. Although designing comprehensive quality system policies and procedures at the department level would appear to be the logical approach in the right direction, precision & accuracy may not be easy to achieve due to various factors.

An interdisciplinary approach would be mandatory to formulate effective treatment plans to resolve the pressing problems in medical science, particularly cancer management.

References

1. Lorenz EN (1963). Deterministic non periodic flow. J Atmos Sci 20: 130-141.

2. Baish JW, Gazit Y, Berk DA, Nozue M, Baxter LT, et al (1996). Role of tumor vascular architecture in nutrient and drug delivery: an invasion percolation based network model. Microvasc Res 51: 327-346.

3. Dey P (2010). Cell modelling and simulation: Fantasy to fact. Bull Med Edu Res 42: 170-176.

4. omita M, Hashimoto K, Takahashi K, Shimizu S, Matsuzaki Y (1999). E-cell: Software environment for whole cell simulation. Bioinformatics 15:72-84.

5. Dey P (2006). Chromatin remodelling, cancer and chemotherapy. Curr Med Chem 13: 2909-2919.

6. Joshi A, Cao D (2010). TGF-beta signalling, tumor microenvirnment and tumor progression: The butterfly effect. Front Biosci 15:180-194.

7. Salto-Tellez M (2007). A case for integrated morphomolecular diagnostic pathologists. Clin Chem 53:1188-1190.

Quality by
design concept

Quality by
design concept

Quality is a pervasive term which is often overused and seldom achieved. Dr Walter Shewhart invented the statistical control chart in 1930s [1] which was utilized by the United States during world war-II the United States along with basic quality control methods to produce military supplies in large quantities cheaply, but with good quality.

In manufacturing, quality is a measure of excellence or a state of being free of defects, deficiencies, and significant variation, brought about by the strict and consistent adherence to measurable and verifiable standards to achieve uniformity of output that satisfies specific customer or user requirement.

ISO 8402-1986 standard defines quality as "the totality of features and characteristics of a product or service that bears its ability to satisfy stated or implied needs."

In manufacturing, one typically adds price or cost into the expectation of quality. However, in medicine, price must be accorded diminished weightage in consideration of quality. According to American National Standards Institute, the definition of quality, accepted by the CAP (College of American Pathologists), is "The totality of features and characteristics of a product or service that bear on its ability to satisfy given needs." Some have defined quality as "Conformance to specification", others have suggested that quality is meeting or exceeding customer expectations. Therefore quality measures needs to be customized [2]. According to ISO 9001 definition; it is set of agreed standards that provide guidelines for a Quality Management System.

In January 2003, the International Organization for Standardization (ISO) published the world's first harmonized clinical laboratory practice standard. Since its publication this standard has gained rapid and widespread acknowledgement and adaptation in many countries. In 2007, the second edition of ISO 15189 was published, with intent to align it further with ISO 17025 [3]. Then how do we define quality in surgical pathology? One major accreditation body, the Joint Commission on Accreditation of Healthcare Organizations (JCAHO), calls for incorporating comparison of organizational performance with that of others, so-called benchmarking of performances [4]. In other words, how does one know that one is as good as one says and what can one learn by comparing oneself with others in competition or even the best in other unrelated business.

The Institute of Medicine (IOM) quality metric defined 6 domains of quality: safety, effectiveness, efficiency, timeliness, equity, and patient centeredness [5]. To accomplish this, basic notions such as quality and product must be defined and understood. Elements of quality that are important in generation of the end product i.e. surgical pathology report include accuracy, timeliness, reproducibility, and completeness. The aim of quality should focus on measuring the complete process from the clinician's perspective.

The entire process of Quality Assurance and Improvement (QA&I) should focus on the process of product generation (surgical pathology report) and product impact (customer or clinician satisfaction). Most would agree that it is easy to define product quality rather than product impact. Figure 1 shows a diagrammatic relation between product requirement (accuracy, timeliness, reproducibility, and completeness) in having appropriate characteristics (clinician satisfaction and patients safety). The existence of relationships between requirements and characteristics makes statements about the quality of product (surgical pathology report).

In surgical pathology, perhaps the worst consequence of poor quality reporting is the inevitable negative outcome resulting from misinformation that may be acted on by the clinician. Some of these reports may be brought to the laboratory's notice, having somehow escaped laboratory attention and fortunately identified by clinical personnel before wreaking any havoc. Nevertheless, these types of errors are quite damaging not only to the laboratory's reputation but also to the clinician's future confidence in the laboratory.

The major product in surgical pathology, that of a diagnosis, results from numerous complex, often manual, sequential processes with interim work products and many human hand-

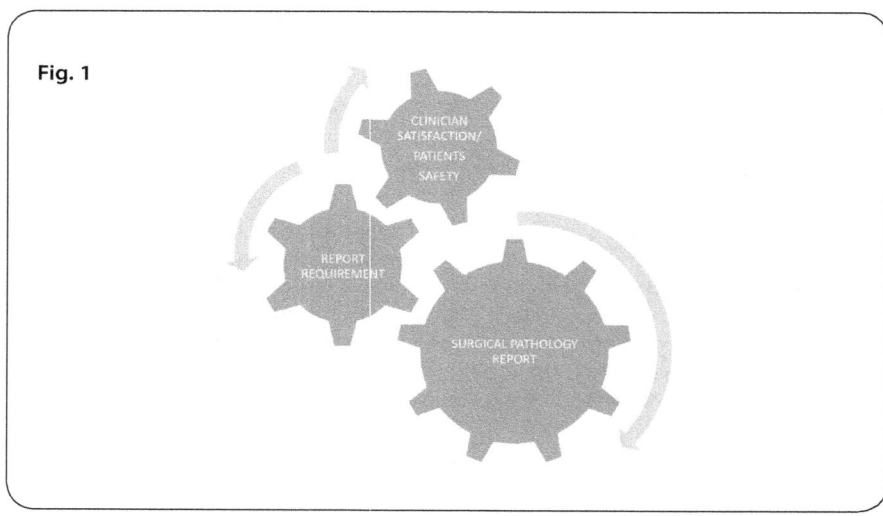

Fig. 1

off points [6]. One should focus on quality product by redesigning, simplifying, and eliminating processes that may have accumulated or been adopted over the years without much thought to efficiency or effectiveness. This quality by design, is nothing but our ability to modify system processes that enhance diagnostic accuracy, information content and completeness as well as timeliness of reporting with reproducibility.

References

1. Best M, Neuhauser D (2006) Walter A Shewhart, 1924, and the Hawthrone factory. Qual Saf Health Care 15: 142-143.

2. Nakhleh RE (2006) What is quality in surgical pathology? J Clin Pathol 59: 669-672.

3. Kawai T (2010) History of ISO 15189 and its future perspective. Rinsho Byori 58: 64-68.

4. Radecki RP, Sitting DF (2011) Application of electronic health records to the Joint Commission's 2011 National Patient Safety Goal. JAMA 306: 92-93.

5. Raab SS, Grzybicki DM (2010). Secondary case review Methods and Anatomic Pathology Culture. Am J Clin Pathol 133: 829-831.

6. Zarbo RJ (2000) The oncologic pathology report. Quality by design. Arch pathol lab Med 124:1003-1010.

Pre-analytic
phase

Pre-analytic
phase

Pre-analytical phase is multifactorial and involves many individuals outside the laboratory. In addition, as the traditional morphological classification is giving way to a newer molecular based classification, the goal is to educate the biomedical community in an effort to improve the quality of RNA that can be recovered from formalin-fixed, paraffin-embedded (FEPE) tissue [1].

In the pre-analytical phase of test cycle, several elements may be monitored including patient satisfaction with collection process, trained professional staff in specimen collection & transport.

Table 1. Gives list of pre-analytical improvement monitors.

Table 1. Pre-analytic improvement monitors	
Directly related to Laboratory	Indirectly related to laboratory
• Specimen fixation • Specimen delivery • Specimen identification • Grossing • Tissue processing • Tissue embedding • Cutting section • Staining, Mounting & Labelling	• Filling requisition form • Adequacy of clinical history with differential diagnosis • Image study reports • Biopsy procedure & primary fixation • Orientation marks for specimen

Specimen collection

The first steps in the process of sample handling are challenging to control, but significantly impact the quality of the specimen. These include time of anaesthesia administration, ligation of vessels, and specimen removal from the patient [2]. These factors cannot be strictly controlled because they influence patient care; however, a detailed recording of these times are an important metric of tissue quality as they affect the quality of the resultant biomolecules, if not cytomorphology directly. The most commonly described impact on tissue quality is the "warm ischemia time" from when the blood supply is ligated until the specimen is received by the pathologist for procurement. This time varies from minutes to hours depending on organs, the surgical approach, the surgeon, nursing staff, and standard operating procedures of the institution [3]. The magnitudes of these changes are poorly understood. All protocols should include the recording of the times for administration of anesthesia, ligation of the vascular supply, and removal of specimen from the patient's body. These times should be included as record submission of the surgical specimen to the pathology department. For biopsies, time of specimen removal should be recorded and communicated to the pathology department.

Specimen labelling

Labelling errors can result in inappropriate therapy or withholding of therapy in patients with unrecognized malignancies. Labelling errors may be detected by laboratory staff, pathologist or a clinician. Labelling errors detected before causing harm or inconvenience to patients are frequently designated as "near misses." [4]

Identification errors involving surgical specimens may involve misidentification of a patient or the patient's specimen or the site from which the specimen was obtained.

Specimen labelling errors within the laboratory can occur at several points of specimen processing. Within the gross room, specimen containers can be paired with cassettes labelled with an incorrect case number (wrong patient) or an incorrect part number (wrong site). In the histology laboratory, cassettes at the cutting station can end up paired with incorrectly pencil-labelled slides (wrong patient or site), or a correctly pencil-labelled slide can have the wrong paper label applied (wrong patient or site).

A surgical pathologist may pick up an incorrect slide and dictate a report with incorrect diagnosis for the patient's laboratory data being reviewed. Errors may also occur during transcription when dictations are transcribed to the wrong report number and patient [5].

Identification of errors fall into 2 categories represented by patient identification errors and specimen identification errors. In patient identification error, a specimen is labelled with the incorrect patient name or identification number. In a specimen identification error, a specimen is misidentified as to site of origin or time of collection but the specimen is correctly associated with correct patient name or identification number.

Identification errors can be classified as pre-analytic, analytic, and post-analytic. All 3 types are of concern to pathologist reputation. Pre-analytic or "clinical" errors can be addressed by standardization of specimen collection process and feedback to clinical staff. Only the analytical errors are directly addressable by laboratory professionals and surgical pathologists. The majority of routine practices for the identification of labelling and specimen identification errors probably underestimates the frequency of occurrence of such errors, and may go undetected [4].

Specimen fixation

The manner in which the specimen is prepared has a dramatic impact on the results. The failure to appreciate and standardize these steps poses problems for both the pathologist & researcher who works with the resultant RNA. The fixation step entails three elements: thickness of tissue, volume of fixative, and time. Failure to optimize all 3 of these elements can result in either underfixation or overfixation of the tissue. Both overfixation and underfixation result in degradation of the specimen after paraffin infiltration, and they hinder correct diagnosis by the pathologist by altering the histomorphology and immunoreactivity [6].

Formalin penetrates tissue at an average rate of 1mm/hour, but this rate can vary depending on tissue type. Standard fixation times are a minimum of 5 hours for needle and endoscopic biopsy specimens and 12 or more hours for sections from larger specimens. These times are required for complete fixation of the specimen. There is unjustified pressure to decrease the time from when tissue is removed until its final diagnosis, which puts the quality of histomorphoogical diagnosis at risk. Reports have described microwave and ultrasound fixation with a variety of fixatives to speed up the fixation of tissue [7].

Grossing

Grossing can contribute to prevention of erroneous specimen identification. The classical pattern of grossing is:

1. handle one specimen at a time;
2. match the requisition form with the container and the processing cassette;
3. double-check the identity of the specimen during dictation.

If the biopsies contain many parts, they should be lined up to check completeness of the case with all possible discrepancies in specimen identification. However, the principle of processing every part of the specimen as a separate entity must be honoured. Although practice sometimes makes correction to this general rule, every grossing person realises that violation of this "grossing central dogma" is dangerous and can lead to a specimen mix-up.

Although some institutions do not use dictation while grossing, it is a commonly accepted practice. Dictations must include, with clear pronunciation, the surgical number, the patients name, and specific identifiers on the container (number, site, content, etc).

Frozen section grossing is prone to specimen misidentification by specifics of the processing. The frozen section area is especially vulnerable if the specimens arrive simultaneously from different patients or as parts of the same patient's specimen, but in bulk. Details of the grossing table configuration are very important for preventing specimen mix-up. Unfortunately, sometimes the grossing person may grab a wrong container or processing cassette. Additional specimen identification on the cassette is common practice.

Defining laterality, type of specimen, or type of procedure sometimes can be useful not only for embedding orientation but act as a safeguard in preventing specimen mix-up. The grossing person must confirm or correct the identifier placed during accession. This is a very important part of preventing specimen misidentification.

The next step, with digital imaging in grossing pathology, can be an additional in preventing erroneous specimen identification. The pathologist would see on the screen not only the specimen's identification documents but actual specimen features (shape, color, size, etc.). Histology information must be entered into the computer by the grossing person, who solely knows all details of the specimen, by using the barcoded requisition forms as the main document.

Another perspective might be an interface between electronic medical records, anatomic information system and a specimen bar-coding system. This would enable tracking a specimen's surgical number, grossing cassettes, embedded blocks, and even microscopic slides during processing cycles. The break in sequence of the surgical numbers or parts of the specimen, double numbers, unexplainable discrepancies between the colour of the cassette according to log, are all safeguards in preventing specimen misidentification [8].

Tissue processing

The process of embedding tissue with paraffin impairs the recovery of biomolecules but appears to have less impact on their quality, as determined by the process of handling and fixation [9]. General recommendation is that detailed records of processing procedures be maintained. Details about the times, temperatures, presence of vacuum and instrument type, as well as the reagent should be included. Accelerated tissue processing protocols require adequate studies to measure their impact on biomolecule recovery and stability. Reagent quality and replacement should be monitored. Studies comparing alternative reagents and processing conditions should be carried out and reported.

The general processing steps include sequential dehydration from an aqueous environment to an alcohol environment (most often ethanol), subsequent replacement by xylene (or xylene substitute) in a process referred to as clearing, and replacement of xylene with paraffin (impregnation). Typically, this process is completely automated, but it lacks standardization and depends on the instrumentation, specimens, and reagents used. Quality of reagents, time, and temperature are sure to impact sample integrity [2].

The duration for complete process can vary from less than 4 hours to more than 12 hours. In general, needle biopsies and bloody specimens should be incubated conservatively, whereas fatty specimen can be processed for longer than average. It is crucial that reagents be of high quality and be replaced on a regular basis. The alcohols and xylenes used in processing become diluted with carry-over from prior steps; as a result, tissue processed at a later time may not be completely dehydrated. The impact of time is similar to that of poor quality exhausted reagents. It is essential that tissue be completely dehydrated during processing, as residual water will not be replaced by paraffin, thus making the tissue susceptible to degradation [2]. The mechanism is probably related to incomplete coagulation of proteins; as a result, water gets trapped within the tissue.

Data concerning alternative reagents and a comparison to the common protocols are lacking. Controlled studies of alternative alcohols and clearing agents have not been carried out for the recovery of nucleic acids. Studies on protein suggest that differences do exist that require modification of downstream protocols.

Embedding and sectioning

The pathologist may guide embedding by notching or inking one or several surfaces of the specimen and providing a "map" in accompanying paperwork that indicates whether these should be placed face-down, face-up, or in parallel with the lateral aspects of cassettes. The embedding step is a potential source of great irritation (and medico-legal liability) for the pathologist if it is done by an inexperienced or careless laboratory worker. Small biopsy specimens that are oriented improperly cannot be interpreted microscopically, necessitating that the block be re-melted and re-embedded. This takes time, and in the process of facing the poorly oriented specimen for preparation of initial sections, valuable tissue may be lost [10].

The paraffin used in impregnation and embedding varies and is chosen to meet the demands of the individual laboratory. Paraffin waxes have different melting points and textures that impact the sectioning characteristics of the final blocks. Not only are a diversity of paraffins used, their exact compositions are often proprietary and/or contain beeswax of marked variation [11]. Synthetic paraffins with low melting temperatures (55-63°C) are typically used in the United States and Western Europe. These formulations may contain latex, dimethyl sulfoxide, and proprietary 'plasticizers' that modify texture and malleability. Beeswax, containing pollen and other contaminants, is routinely used in Eastern Europe, Africa, and South America to modify the melting temperature and improve the malleability of poor-quality paraffin. These interfere with the recovery of biomolecules [12]. The use of higher melting temperature paraffin results in decreased and inadequate de-paraffinization and reduction in the amount of nucleic acids recovered [13]. Low-melting-temperature paraffin is recommended for impregnation of tissue. The type of paraffin should be recorded. Avoid use of a additive such as beeswax.

Histo-microtomy is a seemingly straightforward process, representing the cutting of serial paraffin-embedded sections with tissue microtome. Nevertheless, this technique has many hidden traps that relate to proper maintenance, calibration, and orientation of cutting blades; preparation for paraffin blocks; and dexterity of the technologist. Microtome blades that are dull loose or nicked will produce "chatter" or "venetian blind" artefacts in tissue sections. In addition, the "clearance angle" (angle between the tissue block and the microtome knife) is crucial to good technique. It should be approximately 3-8°. If the angle is too narrow, alternately thick and thin sections are cut, or they are folded on themselves [10]. An excessive clearance angle causes chattered or otherwise hideous sections and may preclude the ability of the technologist to obtain a tissue ribbon. Even worse are the effects of loose microtome blades or tissue blocks in microtome chuck. These deficiencies may shatter the paraffin block entirely or deeply groove the tissue specimen. A block that is mounted crookedly in the microtome chuck will produce irregular ribbons or cause individual sections in the ribbons or cause individual sections in the ribbon to break free from one another. Warm blocks will yield wrinkled ribbons or cause successive sections to anneal to one another. In addition failure to moisten the surface of blocked tissue suitably before cutting will yields an excessive number of knife marks or fragmented sections. Another problem that is sometime seen at this step is tendency for ribbons to "fly" onto the knife blade. This is result of static electricity between the wax or tissue and metal blade, and also may be avoided by slightly moistening the knife and block surface before each ribbon is prepared.

Mounting

The temperature of water bath at the cutting station should be cut at 5-10 °C below the melting point of the embedding wax. If it is too hot, desiccated-looking sections will result; in contrast, cool floatation baths produce excessive wrinkling of the tissue. The ribbons must not be left in the bath for more than 1or 2 minutes, or else will result in spurious over hydration of the tissue. This effect simulates the appearance of oedema fluid microscopically. One of the most dangerous of all mistakes in the histology laboratory can take place when mounting sections from floating baths. Friable tissue may "shred" small fragments that float free on the surface of the water, and these may be inadvertently picked up when mounting slides from subsequently processed unrelated cases. Derisively known as "floaters," these rogue pieces of tissue commonly cause agonizing interpretive problems for the pathologist [10]. An alternative source of floater-type artefacts is the "tongue blade metastasis," wherein tissue adheres to a wooden applicator stick that is used to float successively prepared ribbons from two different cases.

Conclusion

As morphological classifications are gradually being replaced by molecular classification, it has become imperative to preserve & recover nucleic acids. The final product of quality is enhanced by better defining the processes, setting specifications, and approaching tissue as an analyte for molecular analysis [10]. One should encourage a standardized approach for reporting & documenting pre-analytic indicators. Inclusion of these in the checklist of final report will further enhance accountability. The biomedical community will benefit from additional recommendations based on research results demonstrating the quality of nucleic acids recovered from FFPE tissues. In future one can anticipate that the body of knowledge on this important topic of molecular analysis will continue to grow.

References

1. Hewitt SM, Fraser LA, Yanxiang C, Richard CC, Maureen C, et al. (2008) Tissue handling and specimen preparation in surgical pathology. Issues concerning recovery of nucleic acids from formalin-fixed, paraffin-embeded tissue. Arch pathol Lab Med 132:1929-1935.

2. NCCLS (1999) quality assurance for Immunocytochemistry. Approved guidelines. Wayne, Pa:NCCLS;1999. NCCLS document MM4-AC.

3. Dash A, maine IP, Varambally S (2002) Changes in differential gene expression because of warm ischemia time of radical prostatectomy specimens. Am j pathol 161: 1741-1748.

4. Valenstain PN, Sirota RL (2005). Identification errors in pathology and laboratory medicine. Clin Lab Med. 24: 979-996.

5. Layfield LJ, Anderson GM (2010). Specimen labelling errors in surgical pathology: an 18-months experience. Am J Clin Pathol 134: 466-470.

6. De Marzo AM, Fedor HH, Gage WR (2002) Inadequate formalin fixation decreases reliability of p27 immunohistochemical staining: probing optimal fixation time using high-density tissue microarrays. Hum Pathol 33:756-760.

7. Chu WS, Furusato B, Wong K, (2005) Ultrasound-acelerated formalin fixation of tissue improves morphology, antigen and mRNA preservation. Mod Pathol 18:850-863.

8. Demenstein IB (2008). Root cause analysis of specimen misidentification in surgical pathology accession and grossing. Labmedicine 39:497-502.

9. Goldstein NS, Hewitt SM, taylor CR, Yaziji H, and the Members of Ad-Hoc committee on Immunohistochemistry standardization (2007). Recommendations for improved standardization on immunohistochemistry. Appl Immunohistochem Mol Morphol 15: 124-133.

10. Mark RW, Mills NC, Willium KB (2008). Tissue procurement, Processing, and staining techniques. In: Mark RW edidtor. Diagnostic Histochemistry. Cambridge university press. Pp. 1-27.

11. Fricain JC, Rouais F, Dupuy B (1996). A two-step embedding process for better preservation of soft tissue surrounding coral implants. J biomed Mater Res 33: 23-27.

12. Fergenbaum JH, Garcia-Closas M, Hewitt SM, Lissowska J, Sakoda LC, et al. (2004) Loss of antiginicity in stored sections of breast cancer tissue microarray. Cancer Epidemiol Biomarkers Pre. 13:667-672.

13. Chung J-Y, Braunschweig T, Hewitt SM (2006). Optimization of recovery of RNA from formalin-fixed, paraffin- embedded tissue. Diagn Mol Pathol 15:229-236.

Analytical
phase

Analytical
phase

A pathologic diagnosis is the result of a complex series of activities, mastered by the pathologist. Many elements culminate in a diagnosis, including gross dissection and section, embedding, histological sectioning, possible other ancillary studies, and microscopic interpretation. Most critical in this phase is the act of diagnosis itself (Other analytic indicators are depicted in Table 1).

Error-reduction initiatives should target the cognitive component of interpretation error including the implementation of standardized diagnostic criteria, educational initiatives, and the development of redundant systems [1]. Diagnostic interpretation errors may be classified into the categories of slips and mistakes, and studies of cognition have helped to define some error types.

Table 1. Analytic Indicators.

S.No	
1.	Intra-operative Frozen section – permanent section concordance
2.	Histology and gross room monitors • Block labelling errors • Slide labelling errors • Slide quality • Technical skills of histo-technicians
3.	Immunohistochemistry • Frequency of repeat slides • Annual inventory of antibodies and frequency of use • External validation of selected antibodies • Technical skills of technician
4.	Others • Interpersonal relation between laboratory staff • Ancillary study monitors (FISH, EM, Other molecular studies) • Management's commitment to quality

The root cause of interpretation errors generally includes a cognitive failure in conjunction with upstream failures or with system failures. For example, poor- quality specimen may be over-interpreted or under-interpreted, and latent system problems may include pathologist overwork, lack of experience, lack of appropriate redundant systems, etc. The accuracy of the final diagnosis is a measure of the effectiveness of all of these sequential steps. Unfortunately a medico-legal system often ignores system problems and focuses on individual culpability, which is a contrary approach to improving safety systems.

An understanding of the diagnostic process from a theoretical perspective will benefit pathology as a science and as a medical speciality because it provides the basis for under-standing diagnostic variations and discrepancies [2]. The diagnostic process can be viewed as a problem solving strategy. In resolving the problems presented by the case, the pathologist must elaborate an action plan, contemplating four different domains: cognitive, communica-tive, normative, and medical conduct.

Cognitive domain

Pathologists use cognitive process, such as perception, attention, memory, and search, to collect data from the case, including macroscopic and microscopic findings and clinical or radiological information. The process of thinking is consciously guided in the direction of solving problem. Metacognitive skills include planning the way to approach a task, being aware of internal or external distracting stimuli, evaluating progress toward task completion, and maintaining motivation until the task has been completed [3].

When looking at a histologic slide, the pathologist can make a diagnosis, based on a strategy called pattern recognition. Pattern recognition is the realization that the histologic picture conforms to a previously learned picture of the disease. Multiple strategies are employed by pathologists to arrive at a diagnosis similar to their clinical counterparts [4].

Another strategy is called multiple branching or arborisation. In this, there is progression of the diagnostic process down one of a large number of potential, preset paths, by a method in which the response to each diagnostic inquiry automatically determines the next inquiry to be carried out and which, ultimately leads to the correct diagnosis. The algorithm must spelled out in its entirety, before the case arrives, and must include all relevant findings or clues, linking them by pathways that represent the idealized diagnostic process of the expert pathologist.

In exhaustive strategy, the pathologist accumulates all possible data (scrutinizes all the sections, reviews all available clinical data and x-ray, evaluates special stains and immunohistochemistry slides) and proceeds to the second stage of searching for the diagnosis. With experience the pathologist may resort to using short cuts. However, every now and then, the exhaustive strategy may reappear, to aid in ruling out remote diagnostic possibilities, to justify a delay in sign-out while the pathologist considers other relevant points, or to establish rapport with the patients, the clinician, or a referring pathologist in a consulting case.

The hypothetical and deductive strategy comprises 2 elements: hypothesis creation and hypothesis verification. Hypothesis creation is a highly individualistic process and depends on mastery of the dynamic models of structure, function, and response to stimuli that comprise the knowledge from basic science disciplines, such as anatomy, biochemistry, physiology, genetics, basic pathology, and microbiology, as well as clinical medicine, surgery, and dermatology, among others. The second element, hypothesis verification, is a mastery of selection, acquisition, and interpretation of pathologic and para-pathologic data that will best shorten the list of hypothesis.

According to reviews by Foucar [5,6] decision making is an immature scientific field, and it slips into poorly defined, almost transcendental factors, such as intuition, flair, luck, gut impression, and others, which might be related to an implicit or tacit knowledge that pathologists use in making diagnoses, but which are formally expressed. According to him, the pathway to this scientific approach is to progress toward evidence-based medicine. Although not conforming to many of the best standards, the pathologic diagnosis, more often than not, is considered a gold standard to which other standards are compared.

Communicative domain

The written report is a conglomeration of relevant communicative activities like receiving adequate clinical or surgical information, conversing with the clinician or patient, preparing a case for presentation or publication, and image documenting. The nature of warrants and backings will determine the acceptability and certainty of the pathological conclusions. Even if sensitivity and specificity statistics (as well as likelihood ratios and predictive positive and negative values) were to be available for every possible pathologic finding in relation to a diagnosis, such external evidence could never replace individual, pathologic expertise. Put into the context of the dispute between individuality and standardization, the pathologist individually has to choose which standards must be applied in a given case. The available evidence does not always necessitate a particular conclusion; in most cases, the evidence provides some degree of confidence, not absolute certainty. Both the certainty of the scientific knowledge in pathology and the firm conviction of a beyond-a-doubt diagnosis rest on the reasons the pathologist can adduce in refuting objections against them. Previous experience serves as a warrant in an argument. In a particular case, the idea of the objectivity of the histologic perception does not ensure the truth of the corresponding diagnosis; instead, it represents only one instance of an experience in the diversity of its possible interpretations.

In the absence of (and sometimes despite of) good quality research data, pathologic reasoning may be guided by medical heuristics. Of course, medical heuristics may be passed from pathologist to pathologist, in training activities, consultations, books, and meetings, and they form part of background knowledge that pathologist use to make diagnosis, but they are not usually reflected on or made explicit.

Heuristics will always be useful in activating hypotheses, but as anatomic pathology advances as a science, their use is expected to decrease as morphologic findings and molecular techniques are established as more reliable warrants authorizing diagnostic conclusions. Thus argument is useful because it helps to make explicit medical reasoning [7].

Because there are grey zones in medical practice, uncertainty should be clearly acknowledged. This might be a source of considerable epistemological and ethical tension [8].The validity of a pathologic report, depends on 2 conditions:

1. it must be grounded in experience, meaning that it is not dissonant with experience; and
2. the statement must hold up against all counterarguments, i.e. it must be discursively recoverable [9].

A pathologic report, to reach consensus, must be intelligible, must have normative rightness, must not raise doubts about the pathologist's sincerity, and its propositional content must be validated as truth.

Normative domain

As with every human action that has meaning, pathology is driven by rules and norms. The instrumental action is governed by technical rules, which are based on empirical knowledge and which can be proved to be correct or incorrect. The purposive, rational action is governed by strategies (rules of rational choice), which are based on analytic knowledge and which are derived from preference rules and decision-making procedures. Classification schemes should be, as much as possible, based on strategic rules, and the decision to choose which classification is most appropriate for a given case relies on the objectives we have in mind when classifying. The communicative action is governed by social norms that define reciprocal expectations and that must be accepted by at least 2 acting subjects. Whereas the effectiveness of technical rules and strategies depends on the validity of empirically true or analytically correct propositions, the validity of social norms is ensured by inter subjective recognition that is based on consensus or mutual understanding.

Failure to follow proven technical rules or correct strategies may result in lack of success. Learning the rules of instrumental and purposive, rational actions strengthens the pathologist's skills and enables him or her to make diagnoses or, in Murphy's [10] view, to become the medical consultant. Acting in conformity to the norms of communicative action depends on motivations.

Three kinds of rules must be followed (to instrumental action, rational action, and communicative action), with different consequences if they are disrespected [11]. Such rules guide actions that are not opposed to each other; instead, they are complementary and relevant to pathologic practice.

Medical conduct domain

The actions that should be, or are expected to be, carried out by pathologist and the clinician have to be evaluated before the final diagnosis is signed out. The pathologist must clearly know the consequences of a diagnosis in the management of a case, and the report should make clear both the diagnosis and the expected conduct derived from it. The pathologist is technically responsible for the diagnostic interpretation he or she makes. This responsibility is linked to the medical conduct consequent on the diagnosis. As a practicing medical specialist, the pathologist is assumed to be acquainted with the practical implications of his or her diagnoses, thereby admitting responsibility for the actions resulting from them. Medical conduct questions may guide diagnosis and may also contribute to variation, as in the case of a pathologist who feels more comfortable, and therefore more liberal in diagnosing an endometrial curettage specimen from a women in her 50s or older.

Conclusion

Most clinicians see the diagnosis as an instance of problem solving. In the interval between receiving a specimen and signing out a report, the pathologist executes a series of actions and operations. Before proceeding to the actions related to diagnosis, the pathologist should elaborate a plan of action for the problematic case. The implicit knowledge in pathology, comprising many of the tasks involved in diagnosis, involves an interaction among different domains. In a diagnostic task, the:

1. cognitive capability to recognize a histologic finding and to establish a conclusion must be integrated with
2. the communicative ability to appropriately describe and interpret findings and to provide adequate warrants to a conclusion, with
3. obedience to appropriate normative guidelines, and
4. to evaluate the whole task with respect to the conduct that may be instituted as a consequence to the diagnosis.

This know-how in pathology aids in the solution of the case, even if a diagnostic label cannot be applied. When such situation occurs, the pathologist is expected to present a communication stating the facts that precluded a final diagnosis, to follow adequate rules, and also, to propose a managerial approach to the case. The end result "pathology report" should originate in the interest and respect for the patient, and the clinician, as well as other pathologists.

References

1. Raab SS, Grzybicki DM (2010). Qualiy in cancer diagnosis. Ca cancer J Clin 60:139-165.

2. Pena GP, Andrade-filho SA (2009). How does a pathologist make a diagnosis? Arch Pathol Lab Med 133: 124-132.

3. Pena GP, Andrade-Filho JS (2006). Implicacoes cognitivas, filosoficas e educativas do trabalho do patologista. Rev Bras Educ Med. 30:76-86.

4. Sackett DL, Haynes RB, Guyatt GH, Tugwell P (1991). Clinical diagnostic strategies. In: sackett DI, Haynes RB, Guyatt GH, Tugwell P, Editors. Clinical epidemiology. A basic science for Clinical Medicine. 2nd ed. Boston, mass: Little, brown and Co;pp 3-18.

5. Foucar E (1996). Diagnostic decision-making in surgical pathology In: Weidner N, editor. The difficult diagnosis in surgical pathology. Phildelphia, Pa: WB Saunders; pp1-10.

6. Foucar E (2001). Diagnostic decision-making in anatomic pathologist. Am J Clin pathol.21-33.

7. Upshur REG, Cloak E (2003). Argumentation and evidence. Theor Med. 24: 283-299.

8. Pellegrino ED (1999). The ethical use of evidence in medicine. Eval health Prof. 22: 33-43.

9. Habermas J. (2001)Tecrias de la verdad . In: Habermas J, editor. Teoria de la Accion Comunicativa: Complementos y Estudio Previos. 4th ed. Madrid, Spain: catedra; pp 113-160.

10. Murphy WM (2002). The evolution of the anatomic pathologist from medical consultant to information specialist. Am J Surg Pathol 26:99-102.

11. Habermas J (2001). Lecciones sobre una fundamentacion de la sociologia enterminos de teoria del lenguaje. In: Habermas J, editor. Teoria de la Accion Comunicativa: Complementos y Estudios Previos; 4th ed. Madrid, Spain: Catedra, 2001: 19-158.

Standardization of
immunohistochemistry

Standardization of
immunohistochemistry

From the beginning there has been concern relating to the relatively poor reproducibility of immunohistochemical (IHC) method as applied to formalin-fixed paraffin embedded (FFPE) tissue sections, reproducibility on a day to day basis within a single laboratory, and reproducibility among different laboratories. In recent years these concerns have, if anything increased and thelack of 'standardization' is now recognized as a major impediment to basic research, clinical trials, and direct patient care.

A 'total test' approach was advocated in 1992 (Tayler 1992), which in essence, embraces all procedures performed to accomplish an immunohistochemistry (IHC) stain, from sample collection to writing a final report [table 1].

Table 1. Process cycle.

S.No	
1.	PREANALYTICAL Test selection Specimen type Acquisition, pre-fixation and transport Fixation, type and total time Processing and temperature
2.	ANALYTICAL Antigen retrieval procedure Selection of 'primary' antibodies Protocol; labelling reagents Reagent validation Control selection Technical training and certification Laboratory certification and QA programs
3,	POST-ANALYTIC Assessment of control performance Description of results Interpretation/ reporting Pathologist, experience and CME specific to IHC

Immunohistochemistry (IHC) is essentially an ELISA method applied to a tissue section. In this respect, when correctly performed, IHC has the potential to perform as reproducible and quantitative tissue based ELISA assay; much more than a simple stain. That the IHC method mostly does not perform to this level reflects faults in the application of the method, specifically inconsistent sample preparation, lack of references or calibration standards, and inadequate validation of reagents [1]. The use of 'Ready to use' (RTU) does not finally solve these problems, but definitely will lead to increased reproducibility and consistency in a practical sense, in large part by forcing the use of external standards, external reagent validation, and defined, extensively tested protocol upon the user laboratory.

Special stains

The first special stains were variations of the basic biological dyes. Specific histochemical stains soon evolved based on the in situ identification of active enzymes within cells by the

application of colorigenic substrates [2]. Many histochemical methods were, however, technically exacting, both in terms of tissue preparation and staining protocol, a situation that led
to recognition of the critical importance of appropriate positive and negative controls for
interpretation of the findings. Although the methods were challenging enough, the reagents
themselves were often poorly characterized and somewhat variable from manufacturer to
manufacturer and lot to lot. However outdated it may seem to the younger generation pathologist, special stains aid in minimizing the differentials. In United States, the Biologic stain
Commission (BSC) was founded in 1944 as a non-profit corporation, achieved considerable
success with regard to biological dyes, but with the advent of immunohistochemistry, special
stain technology has taken a new leap forward, with great opportunities and new challenges
in standardization.

Clinical question and test selection

In the face of the diagnostic conundrum that cannot be resolved by orthodox morphologic
criteria, the pathologist resorts to his lifeline in the form of ancillary techniques. There is also
an important ongoing shift in emphasis in the use of immunohistochemical stains from primary focus on cell and tissue markers as an aid to the recognition and classification of tumors
to the demonstration of cell products, receptors, or oncogenes of possible prognostic value,
and identification of infectious agents in situ [3].

The first option that a pathologist has, which is the more common modus operandi, is
to select stains from a panel that, in the experience of the pathologist, have proven to be of
value in a particular diagnostic area. The second approach uses an algorithm with sequential
panels of selected stains that indroduces a certain degree of logic and throughness into the
process but may compromise the turnaround time due to sequential staining.

For each stain used in a particular case, the pathologist should ask, and answer, the question, "Will a positive / negative result add to the diagnosis?" If the answer is not known in the
field of pathology or to the individual pathologist, then the stain should not be performed,
because it will not add to the diagnostic equation. The huge variety of reagents available for
IHC, and the large number of different vendors, in a way contributes to lack of standardization; almost there is too much choice [4]. A polyclonal antibody or antiserum is produces by
traditional immunization techniques, with 'booster" injections to maximize reactivity against
the target antigen. Such antisera in fact contain many different antibody 'species', having
varying specificity for many antigens, but are effectively enriched for high affinity antibody
molecules that target the antigen of interest (while antibodies to other antigens, to other
antigens, not of interest, are present at low levels, or are of low affinity, or may be selectively
depleted by absorption methods). Monoclonal antibodies, prepared by hybridoma methods,
or by molecular engineering, contain a single 'species' of antibody molecule, where every antibody molecule is identical by idiotype, with a single affinity. Both polyclonal and monoclonal
antibody reagents must be added to the tissue section at an optimal concentration or working dilution, defined as that giving the highest intensity of specific reaction, with the lowest
level of non-specific background staining: i.e. the highest 'signal to noise ratio'.

Specimen aquisition and management

Pathologists have sought to undo some of the adverse affects of formalin fixation either by the use of controlled enzymatic digestion or the antigen retrieval technique [5]. The latter method (sometimes known as heat-induced epitope retrieval or as unmasking) subjects sections to microwave heating in the presence of a retrieval solution that may serve to stabilize or postfix the antigens present. Although vigorous heating in a microwave oven offends basic instincts, the method has contributed to the reproducibility of immunostaining by providing a more uniform presentation of antigens in tissue sections than is otherwise present following inconsistent fixation in formalin. However, one significant caveat has been issued [6] namely that "as different antigen retrieval approaches are explored and propagated, there is a danger that a different procedure, producing varying degrees of restoration of antigenicity, will add yet another variable to the overall process." Unfortunately this warning has come to pass [5]. Clearly, the preference is for anatomic pathologist to adopt more uniform and rigorous procedures for the fixation and processing of tissues, extending from the moment that the specimen is removed from the body to the end of the embedding process, particularly controlling the total time in fixative itself. The pressure for consistency in staining has grown even further because of the increasing focus on prognostic markers, where greater stringency is required [2].

Reagent validation

While choice and validation of reagents are critical issues, by far the most important contributory factor to variable performance of IHC worldwide, as well as in individual laboratories, relates to the 'pre-analytic' phase [7,8]. In this respect the more widespread use of RTUs may have benefit, not solving the problem of standardization, but perhaps contributing to some practical improvement. The laboratory should focus upon selecting the optimal concentration (or working dilution) of primary and secondary reagents, or electing instead to use RTUs with defined detection systems and protocols. It must be stressed that other aspects of the IHC protocol are also of critical importance in achieving consistency, including selection and validation of any antigen retrieval procedure, precision in volume of reagents applied to the slide, choice and pH of dilution buffers, optimized incubation times (at defined temperature), number and effectiveness of wash cycles, and concentration, temperature and incubation time of the chromogen of choice.

There are at least 25 separate steps in a typical IHC assay. All must be optimized and performed in an identical manner, run after run, day after day; and ideally from laboratory to laboratory. In this respect, use of an automated system can greatly enhance reproducibility within a laboratory, whether using concentrated reagents and self optimized detection systems, or RTUs. The use of RTUs has an additional benefit for many laboratories in that it forces standardization of reagents, dilutions, detection systems, and overall protocol among different laboratories using the same system [4]. Internal consistency is more readily achieved with RTUs than with use of concentrated reagents, because of the inherent variability in optimization of the latter among different laboratories. Furthermore, as several laboratories adopt the same RTUs, detection systems and protocols, improved standardization will result, against the remaining major variable of sample preparation.

Use of controls

The proper use of appropriate controls is vital to all IHC assays, and should include a positive control, and a negative control. In practice the positive control is usually a tissue section fixed and processed in similar manner to the test section and known to contain the target molecule, ideally based upon independent assay, but more often based upon presumptive presence of the target molecule derived from knowledge of the literature and prior experience. Positive controls ideally should be selected for giving a range of intensity of reaction, from strong to intermediate to weak; use of tissue containing very high amounts of antigen may lead to selection of optimal working dilutions that fail to detect lower levels of the target antigen found in other (pathological) tissues. The term 'negative' control, covers two control concepts; a 'negative reagent control', typically omitting the primary antibody on a parallel tissue section that otherwise is treated identically, and a 'negative tissue or cell control', typically omitting the primary antibody on a parallel tissue section that otherwise is treated identically, and a 'negative tissue or cell control'. In practice the latter requirement is in most cases fulfilled by identification of non-staining cell types within the test section, that is cells that do not contain the target molecule, and do not, therefore give positive reaction [4].

Analytic skills

The experience and training of the technologist who is performing the stain clearly are critical to this process. One major factor in ensuring reproducibility may be the growth of automation, with the extended capability for consistency and control that is inherent in the automated process. The availability of automated immunostainer has proven overall benefit in many smaller laboratories, if not some larger ones, that do not have the luxury of highly skilled staffs who are experiences in reagent titration and quality control [2].

The interpretation and significance of the finding should be presented in the context of the overall differential diagnosis. Interpretation of the presence of specific positive staining, or lack thereof, is, of course, a complex issue. It is a function of the performance and examination of the proper controls and examination of the proper controls and the experience of the laboratory performing the stains, especially the pathologist responsible for evaluating the stained slides. A second aspect to interpretation relates to the way we arrive at an opinion regarding the significance of a particular set of staining results in relation to diagnosis or prognosis of the patient. Most surgical pathology publications now incorporate immunohistochemical findings to some degree. To keep pace with the relevant literature is a challenge that is impossible to meet in broad perspective. The prototypic Web site, pioneered by Dennis Frisman [9], may provide precedent for the future but suffers from selectivity of content and places great demands on the Web master for maintenance of currency.

Conclusion

There have been several schools of thought as to the reason why IHC 'stains' are difficult to run in a reproducible or consistent manner. If there is a consensus as to the cause of lack of standardization, it is that several reasons conspire together. Resolution of 'pre-analytic' issues (sample preparation, fixation) will require an order of general collaboration hitherto unseen, even should there be agreement as to which new and better fixative to use.

IHC must be performed only with a degree of technical rigor and control that matches any other immunologically based assay of like principle (namely ELISA). Like ELISA, RTUs coupled with proven detection systems, fixed protocols, recommended controls and automation, represent an analogous pathway that can lead to improved levels of reliability and performance of IHC. Collectively, these processes almost certainly will elevate standards, but to a degree they are peripheral to the problem.

References

1. Taylor CR (2006). Quantifiable internal reference standards for immunohistochemistry: the measurement of quantity by weight. Applied immunohisto Mol Morph 14: 253-259.

2. Taylor CR (2000). The total test approach to standardization of immunohistochemistry. Arch Pathol Lab Med 124: 945-951.

3. Taylor CR, Cote RJ (1997). Immunohistochemical markers of prognostic value in surgical pathology. Histol Histopathol 12:1039-1055.

4. Taylor CR(2009). Immunohistochemical standardization and ready- to- use antibodies. In: George LK, Rudbeck L, editors. IHC staining methods. Dako, Northamerica; California. pp 21-28.

5. Shi SR, Cote RJ, Chaiwun B, Young LL, Shi Y, et.al (1998). Standardization of immunohistochemistry based on antigen retrieval technique for routine formalin-fixed tissue sections. Appl Immunohistochem 89-96.

6. Shi SR, Key NE, Kalra KL (1991). Antigen retrieval in formalin-fixed, paraffin embedded tissue: An enhancement method for immunohistochemical staining based on microwave oven heating of tissue sections. J Histochem Cytochem 39:741-748.

7. Taylor CR(2006). Standardization in immunohistochemistry: the role of antigen retrieval in molecular morphology. Biotechnic & Histochemistry. 81: 3-12.

8. Miller RT, Swanson PE, Wick MR (2000). Fixation and epitope retrieval in diagnostic immunohistochemistry: A concise review with practical considerations. Appl Immunohistochem Morphol 8:228-235.

9. Frisman D. Immunohistoquery. Available at: http:/immunoquery.com.

Classification in
surgical pathology

Classification in
surgical pathology

Classification is the activity that allows pathologists to arrange the bewildering morphologic manifestations of disease into comprehensible order. However, in spite of the amazing success of pathology classification, it is apparent to everyone that diagnostic disagreements are common , and that that patients who exactly fit into a diagnostic category often have markedly different disease courses and response to therapy. This has partly led us shift from phenotypic- clinical framework of diagnosis, into phenotypic–molecular-clinical dimension [1].

As a result of this shift, the process leading from pathological diagnosis to therapeutic decision making includes an area of increasing molecular diagnostic complexity that, in most instances, is not directly addressed by surgical pathologists. The future consequence of this trend is clear: conventional surgical pathology will not be less important (the morphological characterization of the disease will always be a starting point of the diagnostic process), but molecular testing, rather than morphological characterization, may provide the decisive information for diagnosis and treatment. It is clear that the pathology classification will undergo substantial changes to include molecular dimension (e.g., Breast malignancies, Leukemias, Brain tumors, etc.), and molecular testing will affect areas of diagnostic decision-making that are currently within the exclusive realm of morphologists [2].

Genetic studies have revealed that there are different pathways to a successful phenotype, and, therefore, "looks like" does not always mean genetically "closely related to" [3,4]. Diagnostic resolution is changing from comparisons of cell size to identification of single nucleotide polymorphisms (variation shared by at least 1% of the target population). However, new molecular technology will replace the microscope based pathologist only if the knowledge produced by this technology is more valuable in clinical setting and more cost effective. Unless political or economic pressures force diagnosis into selected centres of excellence, a classification system can be considered successful only when it can be used correctly in a broad range of practice settings.

Precision and accuracy

Despite the availability of miraculous new tools to assist in classification, pathologists continue to struggle with issues that are analogous to those faced by ancient and more modern taxonomists. Measures of accuracy and precision are two quite different, basic methods of assessing the clinical usefulness of a classification system. Precision is the measure of the degree of intraobserver and interobserver variation in assigning a case to a given diagnostic category, while accuracy is the closeness of the diagnosis to the true clinical state, encompassing such features as clinical manifestations, clinical course, and response to therapy.

It is important to recognize that whether diagnostic agreement is with peer group or with one or more experts, agreement is simply agreement, and no level of agreement transforms precision into accuracy. Accepting agreement is nothing more than a dangerous substitute for accuracy. When objective clinical data such as a distinctive clinical course or a distinctive response to therapy are not available to establish accuracy, pathology precision may have to serve as a surrogate for how the patient feels, functions, or survives [5]. If suppose all pathologists agree with a certain diagnosis on a case, but the biology of the patient's disease does not conform to that of other members of the assigned diagnostic category, the diagnosis is precise but not accurate. In contrast, a diagnostic category that lacks precision cannot be accurate because patients are not assigned to the category in a consistent fashion. So, imprecise categories can exist in the realm of text books or classification schemes, but without precision, they do not exist as a clinical reality.

In a sense, they are pathology fiction, which is a subtype of science fiction. It is only through the possession of diagnostic precision that a theory is transformed into a diagnostic category that can be then studied and clinically defined. A set of rules for diagnosis does not establish a scientific pedigree for a category, because the application of rules to problems is common to both scientific and non-scientific activities. True scientific rules should not be falsifiable, and because they do not require any private interpretation or divine inspiration, should give similar results when used by trained individuals. Most important, there is no standard for judging what level of diagnostic disagreement is clinically acceptable. The centrality of precision to science is highlighted by the annual Ig Nobel Prize ceremony, which showcases work that either "cannot or should not be reproduced"[6].

Types of classification

To understand classification, the pathologist must understand the fundamental distinctions between different types of classification. One important subtype of classification is category assignment. When performing diagnostic category assignment, the pathologist deals with categories that are given, and the rules for sorting are unambiguous and in place. The common denominator of assignment is not that it is simple, but rather that once the diagnostic data is collected, they are unambiguous and lead directly to one diagnosis.

In contrast with category assignment, other types of classification require the pathologist to deal with exceptions or new configuration of data. At one extreme, classification requires that both categories and the rules for assignment be developed from scratch; there are no established assignment rules to violate [7]. At the other end of classification is structured classification, which begins with the acceptance of a set of categories and diagnostic rules. When cases are encountered that do not follow the rules or fit the categories, the pathologist makes modifications in the existing framework.

Pathologists usually are engaged in assignment behaviour but must occasionally switch to structured classification activities when rules must be modified before assigning an unusual case to an existing category. In pathology, as in other branches of science, the truth lies somewhere in sociology and science, Understanding pathology classification requires understanding that these systems are developed through a political process.

What is the best classification?

Epidemiologists will be interested in etiology and epidemiology; pathologists in morphology, postulated normal cellular counterpart, immunophenotype, and genetics; clinicians in prognosis, distinctive responses to therapy, and clinical features. Surgical pathology has remained heavily dependent on experts to provide a gold standard for what is correct and what is incorrect classification assignment. This problem of identifying valid classification gold standards has proven particularly challenging for the speciality in the area of early diagnosis, where links between tissue classification and outcome are increasingly obscured by the murky concepts of predisposition and risk [8,9,10].

Predisposition diagnoses are designed to reduce the incidence of advanced disease in a population, not to predict the specific outcome for an individual patients. When increases in screening sensitivity abruptly presented surgical pathologists with large number of cases with "early" changes of malignancy, the speciality had the stark choice of either admitting that even experts did not really understand the significance of these new lesions flooding into their laboratories or continuing to classify poorly understood lesions as malignancy based on historic diagnostic criteria [5]. A short-term choice to classify lesions of low or uncertain biological potential as carcinoma while things got sorted out would have been understandable because surgical pathology is a field with no foundation in statistics or epidemiology. In the future, diagnostic advances may present the oncopathologist with more examples of clinically healthy individuals found to have a few cells that share some morphologic or molecular features with established malignant cell population [11].

Neither the patient nor the clinician cares whether a tumour forms glands or makes keratin, but both would like information that leads with highest degree of certainty to currently available efficacious therapy, i.e., a patient management-driven classification system. Pathologist rather than being simply a taxonomist, should act as a patient advocate sensitive to the clinical implications of diagnostic categories. However, one finds that in practice, a gold standard that heavily depends on clinical relevance is quite difficult to maintain. In a patient care environment where therapy is either changing or variable from clinician to clinician, clinical relevance can be one more factor adding empty complexity to the classification. Even when largely based on the features of cells, a classification system must acknowledge and accommodate this truth that the task at hand is patient care.

The design of classifications

In the past, individuals introduced, promoted, and defended classification systems, and sometimes there seemed to be more attention paid to documenting priority or jousting with rivals than to documenting either precision or accuracy [12]. Ideally expert group on classification, should be multidisciplinary, should base recommendation on a systematic review of published work, and should explicitly state the rationale and the strength of the evidence that supports each recommendation [13]. Still there could be limitation to classification system; four such important limitations are

1. Data limitations

One of the most basic problems that must be confronted in classification is that the data themselves do not resolve the conflict between lumpers and splitters. The only rational limitation on the splitters is that the number of categories should not exceed the number of cases available for classification. In contrast, the lumpers are limited only by the conceptual problem of having less than one category. When developing classification schemes, one option is to narrowly focus the definition of categories so that do not every case meets the criteria for inclusion is very similar to every other case. However, given the nature of biology, this often either will leave many cases that do not precisely fit the criteria for any category or will require large number of categories with the attendant complexity and imprecision. In contrast, if the criteria for categories are broad, almost every case will find a category "home," but the categories will often contain a very heterogeneous group of patients, essentially defeating the purpose of classification.

2. Self-interest

Like all other aspects of science, classification systems are the products of individuals who have a stake in the outcome of their work. The degree to which a classification system becomes influential contributes directly to the professional status of the individuals involved in the system's development. One mechanism to decrease the importance of self-promotion is to include as participants in the development of classifications a substantial percentage of individuals who are new to the process [5].

3. Consensus

Achieving consensus is as much a social as a scientific process. Since even the best evidence includes elements of uncertainty, consensus conclusion demands judgement. A WHO committee on Histologic typing of tumours included "many years of unsuccessful negotiations and deliberations" according to one of the participants [14]. When consensus is a goal, then lack of consensus is failure. A logical technique to avoid failure is to exclude individuals known to have opinions outside the mainstream or contrary to those of the group organizing the conferences. But this consensus may be a simplification of the current state of knowledge. Those who believe that their input was not given sufficient weight will perceive the consensus committee's conclusion as illegitimate [14].

4. Compliance

How does an expert committee convince thousands of geographically dispersed independent practitioners to adopt the new system? Clinical studies have suggested problems with compliance if there is a lack of an accountability component or if there is a reliance on voluntary change without accompanying incentives [15].

Conclusion

In our opinion, the term "Final Diagnosis" best suits, well written novel scripts rather than a pathology report. The final word should always end with "Impression" or "Opinion" just to accommodate the risk of judgemental error. A disease labelled can perhaps be considered a disease half conquered, but a disease mislabelled is surely a disease that will remain misunderstood. A speciality's weak ties to the scientific method are provided by very slow recognition of error [16].

A classification of each era reveal just how effectively pathologists working at that time were able to separate, precedent, contemporary politics, and superstition from scientific evidence. Ideas should be judged by whether they were reasonable in the historic context in which they were proposed. Successful advances in disease classification are achieved through the evolutionary mechanisms of selection acting on variation.

References

1. Salto-Tellez M (2007). A case for morphomolecular diagnostic pathologists. Clin. Chem. 53:1188-1190.

2. Heffner DK (2001). The end of surgical pathology. Ann diagn Pathol 5: 368-373.

3. Kenrick P (1999). The family tree of flowers. Nature. 402: 358-359.

4. Srinivasan MV (1999). When one eye is better than two. Nature. 399: 305-307.

5. Foucar E (2001). Classification in Anatomic pathology. Am J clin Pathol 116:S5-20.

6. Nadis S (1999). Ig prizes spawn a new generation of Nobels. Nature 401:518.

7. Hand DJ (1997). Construction and Assessment of classification rules. New York, NY: John wiley & Sons. Pp1-20.

8. Evans JS (1999). Reviewer. Calculating the chances. Review of: kammen DM, Hassenzahl DM. Should we risk it? Science. 285:1857.

9. Foucar E (1996). Carcinoma-in-situ of the breast: have pathologists run amok? Lancet 347:707-708.

10. Foucar E. Do pathologist play dice? Uncertainty and early histopathological diagnosis of common malignancies. Histopathology. 31:495-502.

11. Schnittger S, Wormann B, Hiddemann W, (1998). Partial tandem duplications of the MLL gene are detectable in peripheral blood and bone marrow of nearly all healthy donors. Bllod 92: 1728-1734.

12. Dorfman RF (1974). Classification of non-Hodgkin's lymphomas. Lancet. 2: 961-962.

13. Miller J, Petrie J (2000). Development of practice guidelines. Lancet 355:2172.

14. Suster S, Moran CA (1999). Thymoma classification: the ride of the Valkyries? Am J Clin Pathol. 112: 308-310.

15. Smith TJ, Hillner BE (2001). Ensuring quality cancer care by the use of clinical practice guidelines and critical pathways. J Clin Oncol. 19:2886-2897.

16. Platt JR (1964). Strong inference. Science 146:347-353.

Postanalytic
phase

Postanalytic
phase

Post-analytic phase of the test cycle begins with dictation of the gross and microscopic examination and the final diagnosis and includes transcription, report correction, verification, and report delivery [1]. The use of summary checklist has been shown to be very effective in providing more complete reports [2]. TAT is a critical element of quality and usually covers all aspects of the laboratory test cycle. While TAT may be fragmented into smaller components, the total TAT is the only measure by which the clinician or customer will judge the pathology report. Smaller components, however, are important to understand when an intervention is planned to improve the total TAT. Post analytic parameters can be grouped into three indicators:

a. Technical issues related to laboratory
b. Total turnaround time (TAT)
c. Clinician satisfaction and/or complaints (table 1).

Table 1. Postanalytic indicators.

S.No	
1.	Technical issues related to laboratory • Transcription errors • Verification errors • Report delivery errors • Incomplete errors • Diagnostic finding correlation with ancillary studies (IHC, EM, FISH)
2.	Turnaround time (TAT) • Frozen section • Biopsy • Large specimen • Preliminary and final necropsy reports
3.	Clinician satisfaction and / or complaints • Interpersonal relation between clinician & pathologist • Diagnostic accuracy • Frozen section timeliness and accuracy • Report timeliness • Report completeness • Pathologist availability • Recent changes

Customer or clinician satisfaction is probably one of the most important measures of quality because it lends insight into a clinician's perception of the pathology report. While there are many elements that when combined add up to a quality report, clinician satisfaction is also based on the additional factor of expectation [3]. Thus a laboratory may have accurate, timely, and complete reports, yet a clinician may still have the perception of poor quality if they have unrealistic expectations. Therefore, in addition to managing and monitoring all elements of quality, the pathologist must also manage clinician expectations and make sure that they are realistic. Without some effort to obtain clinician feedback, some problems, at least from the clinician's perspective, may never be identified.

Quality assurance consultation

The experience of the pathologist has an impact on the precision of the pathology findings. Pathologists choosing to practice within a distinct sub-speciality acquire a fund of knowledge during fellowship training that extends beyond anatomic and clinical pathology residency training. Additionally, sub-speciality pathologists, when defining their practice exclusively within their area of expertise (accepting specimens limited to their area of speciality) may review significantly greater numbers of cases over a shorter period of times as compared to general pathologist - complementing deeper fund of knowledge with rapidly acquired experience measured in tens to hundreds of thousands of cases.

Within a general pathology setting, an individual pathologist may review a total of 6000 cases each year – distributed among each of the organ systems: 30% gastrointestinal, 25% skin, 20% urologic, 15% breast and gynaecological; and 10% a mixture of the remaining organ systems. That translates to an approximate case experience of 1,800 gastrointestinal; 1,500 skin; 1,200 urologic; 900 breast and gynaecological; and 600 other cases each year. For comparison, experienced gastrointestinal pathologists who selectively practice gastrointestinal pathology may review 10,000 cases each year – with all 10,000 cases gastrointestinal specimen [4]. Interpretive error reduction strategy should be part of quality assurance programme (Table 2).

Table 2. Interpretive error reduction strategies: types of observer redundancy.

- Double-read: general sign-out with intradepartmental consult voluntary, individual diagnostic thresholds mandated by organ, diagnosis, or percent of cases blinded or public review, by individual or panel selected slide or entire case
- Correlation review
- Conference/ Tumour board review
- Extra-departmental consult
- Institutional review (Outside cases)

Effective communication

Evidence supporting the high value of clinician-pathologist communication for planning the best clinical management for patients with malignant disease of all stages may consistently be found in studies evaluating the impact of multidisciplinary conferences (MC) or tumour boards (TB) [5,6]. Consultative discussions among all physicians (including radiologists and pathologists) on the patient care team take place, with a patient management plan as the outcome. The specific activities should include, review of previous radiologic and pathologic test results with review of outside materials by in-house radiologist, pathologist and a multidisciplinary discussion about the diagnostic and management aspects of case.

This enhanced communication among multiple speciality physicians has been shown to result in significant numbers of changes in both the type and stage of reviewed cases. The occurrence of these discussions in cancer centre settings has also shown to positively impact patient receipt of management best practices [7]. Patients should be given opportunity to discuss his/her diagnostic testing and diagnosis with the participating pathologist(s) and radiologist(s) [8]. Therefore, during face to face verbal communication among physician, clinical information also appears to be exchanged, and that exchange contributes to changes in diagnostic and prognostic information, which then may produce changes in patient management. There is a definite positive impact on oncologic diagnostic test accuracy and patient management decisions made in formal, structured forum for interdisciplinary physician-physician communication [7]. No evidence is currently available that describes the impact of individual clinician-pathologist dialogue during routine daily practice on pathologic diagnoses or clinical management plans for patients with malignancies.

Different review methods

1. Subspecialist review method

Many laboratories and healthcare institutes, in an effort to increase quality and reduce diagnostic inaccuracy, have adopted partial or complete sub-speciality pathologist sign-out cases. This distribution and review of cases represents a significant cultural and system change from the general pathologist-driven pathology practice, in which "every pathologist signs out every type of case." Many clinicians accept sub-speciality sign-out, the patient and clinician experience the benefit of pathologists practicing with a limited, but specialized skill set, generally complemented by the use of standardized terminology common to both the pathologist and the clinician specialist. Sub-speciality pathologist review of cases may result in consistent adherence to established diagnostic criteria, pathologist's ability to correlate objective pathologic tissue data with subjective and objective clinical information, and the ability to provide a "common language" to facilitate ease of communication of the pathology report.

2. Consultative review

Consultative review of pathology materials (second opinions) is an essential component of total quality assurance programs in diagnostic surgical pathology and cytopathology [9]. This key aspect in the assurance of patient's safety for tissue-and cytology-based diagnoses is likely to be the most accurate and cost-effective when a program combines:

- Prospective intradepartmental review of cases,
- Retrospective intradepartmental review of diagnoses rendered,
- Selected utilization of inter-institutional second opinions referred to pathologist with sub-speciality expertise within specific organ system and disease categories, and
- Mandatory review of pathology materials in which the diagnosis was reported at external institutions when patients are referred for definitive therapy within the "home" institution [10].

While these components of quality assurance programs may appear "self-evident" or universally accepted, self-reporting surveys of academic and community hospitals demonstrate that each of these measures is performed consistently within the pathology department of only 30% to 65% of institutions [11].

3. Intra-departmental consultation

The elements of quality assurance consultation is most essential within department, institution, or organization can be assessed by compiling and/or requesting specific reports of consultation activities by pathologists; policies to incorporate:
- Mandatory second pathologist review when indicated by current standard of care (any malignancy, high grade dysplasia in Barrett's, any dysplasia in IBD, and others).
- Consensus conference activities within the department to set standards and 'thresholds" for diagnosis. Documenting altered judgemental reports based on clinical findings & patients safety.
- Prospective documented and confidential peer review of challenging cases – recording minor and major discrepancies within the department.
- Retrospective review of 2% of all cases, randomly selected, or selected by organ system for systematic review.
- Inquiries to the pathologist and department:
  1. Which pathologists have subspecialty expertise in which organ system and/or disease? Is this formal or informal training?
  2. Is the intradepartmental consultation directed to pathologists with sub-speciality expertise or distributed among the pathologists in another manner?
  3. What are the rates of minor and major discrepancies among the pathologist?
  4. How are the discrepancies resolved?

4. Extra- departmental (Inter-institutional review)

- Mandatory review of any outside pathology materials upon which a definitive therapy is planned within a referral institution.
- External consultation by sub-speciality pathologists required on no less than 0.5% of all cases. Within a community hospital with 20,000 cases each year, this results in 100 cases for consultation each year; roughly 2 cases per week [4].
- Inquiries to the pathologist and department:
  1. What is the ratio of inter-institutional consultation performed (a) at the request of the patient; (b) at the request of the clinicians; (c) at the request of the treating institution and (d) at the request of the pathologist rendering the original diagnosis?
  2. Does the pathology department utilize a specific set of preferred consultants who are recognized experts within each subspeciality?
  3. Alternately, do the referral cases get "sent to the university," without specifying a consultant pathologist?
  4. What is the rate of diagnostic agreement? Minor disagreement? Major disagreement? With the consulting pathologist?
  5. Are disagreements discussed with "in-house" pathologist? Are his explanations documented?
  6. How are these discrepancies resolved?

Conclusion

Clinical colleagues have two broad expectation from the anatomic pathologist. First is verification of diagnosis. Clinicians expect pathology consultants to have reviewed and correlated previous pertinent diagnostic material and to inform them of clinically important discrepancies or clinical opportunities. The second major expectation is that pathologist will consistently provide information to routinely satisfy clinical needs [12].

In many cases, a clinician wants the result in black or white, which may not be possible with present knowledge of particular disease. Therefore, simplification of the result is sometimes called for, despite all skills and knowledge, the pathologist is expected to know of the art and science behind the pathology report. Documentation of these arts on long run will add value in health care delivery setting and formulating legal boundaries.

Reference

1. Fitzgibbons PL (2005). Post analytic variables: report adequacy and integrity. In: Nakhleh RE, Fitzgibbons PL, editors. Quality management in anatomic pathology: promoting patients safety through systems improvement and error reduction. Northfield: the college of American pathologists, pp 61-65.

2. Branston LK, Greening S, Newcombe RG, et al (2002). The implementation of guidelines and computerized forms improves the completeness of cancer pathology reporting. The CROPS project: a randomized controlled trial in pathology. Eur J Cancer 38: 764-772.

3, Zarbo RJ, Nakhleh RE, Walsh M (2003). Customer satisfaction in anatomic pathology; a College of American Pathologist Q-probes study of 3065 physician surveys from 94 laboratories. Arch pathol lab Med. 127: 23-29.

4. Dahl J (2006). Quality, Assurance, Diagnosis, Treatment, and Patient Care. Patients safety & Quality healthcare. http://www.psqh.com/.

5. Gatcliffe TA, Coleman RL (2008). Tumor board: more than treatment planning- a 1year prospective survey. J cancer Edu. 23: 235-237.

6. Petty JK, vetto JT (2002). Beyond doughnuts: tumor board recommendation s influence patient care. J cancer Edu. 17: 97-100.

7. Raab SS, Grzybicki DM (2010). Quality in cancer diagnosis. Ca Cancer J Clin 60: 139-165.

8. Newman EA, Guest AB, Helvie MA, Roubidoux MA, Chang AE, et al (2006). Changes in surgical management resulting from case review at a breast cancer multidisciplinary tumor board. Cancer. 107: 2346-2351.

9. Tomaszewski JE, Bear HD, Connally JA, Epstein JI, Feldman M, et al. (2000). Consensus conference on second opinions in diagnostic anatomic pathology: Who, what and when. Am J Clin pathol. 114: 329-335.

10. Sarewitz SJ (n.d.) Laboratory accreditation program inspection checklists. College of American pathologist. http://www.cap.org/.

11. Gupta D, Layfield LJ (2000). Prevalence of inter-institutional anatomic pathology slide review: a survey of current practice. Am J Surg pathol. 24: 280-284.

12. Zarbo RJ (2000). The oncologic pathology report. Arch pathol Lab Med124: 1004-1010.

Error taxonomy
and validation

Error taxonomy
and validation

There are four general types of errors, with 3 sub-types in the category of defective interpretation [1].

1. The first subtype is a false negative diagnosis or under call of the extent of severity of a lesion.
2. The second is a false-positive diagnosis or an over-call.
3. The third subtype is misclassification (Table 1).

When error is detected, amendment options include changes in (a) the primary diagnostic characteristics (eg, change from negative to positive, benign to malignant, or inadequate to adequate); (b) the second diagnostic characteristics (eg, tumour grade, stage, margin, or node status); (c) diagnostic reclassification (eg, the fibrosarcoma changed to malignant fibrous histiocytoma in which primary or secondary diagnostic change does not alter the prognostic impact of the classification); (d) patient or specimen re-identification; (e) report of additional specimen sampling that has resulted in the changed report; and (f) other edits of the reports that do not change primary or secondary diagnostic information, patient or specimen identification, or involve specimen characteristics.

Table 1. Common error types in all total test cycle phase.

S.No	
1.	Defective Identification • Patient • Tissue • Laterality (right vs. left) • Anatomic location
2.	Defective Specimen • Lost specimen, inadequate volume, size, gross description, erroneous measurement or extraneous tissue. • Inadequate representativeness/ sampling (tissue, blocks, levels) • Pertinent ancillary diagnostic study not initially done.
3.	Defective report • Erroneous/ missing non-diagnostic information • Dictation/ Typing error • Report delivery • Computer/format, transmission, upload error

4.	Defective Interpretation
	• False negative – Undercall
	• False positive – Overcall
	• Mis-classification: not altering primary or secondary diagnostic characteristics
	   - Primary = Positive/ negative or benign/malignant
	   - Secondary = Grade, stage, margin, ect.

Timing of discovery segregates into those cases detected before sign-out (before case is finalized) and those detected after sign-out (after a report has been produced).

For changes detected before sign-out, four mechanisms are possible: the effect of (a) additional information or material; (b) intradepartmental review before sign-out or double read of the current case ;(c) preparation for presentation at a conference or at review with clinician; and (d) an external consultation.

For the revisions after sign-out, possible mechanisms are: (a) The responsible pathologist's review of a recent case without additional information or material; (b) the responsible pathologist's review of a recent case with additional information or material but without clinical prompting; (c) at preparation or presentation at conference with clinicians (e.g., tumour board); (d) clinician-initiated review or reconsideration of a case; and (e) as the result of an external consultation.

A single classification system cannot adequately fulfil the differing needs of these two purposes. Temporal considerations force a subdivision of the evaluation into an initial assessment at the time of discovery and follow-up assessment after 3 months of discovery. The classification of discrepancies/errors provided in the Royal college of pathologist publication (2006), entitled 'concerns about performance in pathology: guidance for healthcare organizations and pathologists' (Table 2).

Table 2. Terminology.

S.No	
1.	A diagnostic error, which is likely to have a definite influence on clinical management and possible outcome
2.	A misinterpretation or oversight, which has the potential to affect clinical management or outcome
3.	A minor discrepancy of disease categorisation, which is likely to be of little clinical significance.

However, in November 2007, The professional performance panel, submitted recommendations to the professional Standards Unit [2]. The summaries of that proposal were as follows:

Definitions-

- A discrepancy can be defined as a difference of opinion between the original interpretation at review
- A discrepancy can only be considered an error when the discrepancy is confirmed by two independent reviewers
- What is the purpose to evaluate discrepancies?
- Response to an expression of concern about a doctor's performance: to ascertain if there is substance to the concerns about a doctors performances, to identify where these concerns lie and what could be done about these concerns.
- Duty care review: to identify patients whose care may have been sub-optimal with a view to rectify any deficiencies in care. This is usually undertaken when concerns about performances have been established.

Error rates can be heavily influenced by classification system but also interpersonal relation with auditing authority. Performance and art of practice are multifaceted skills acquired and influenced by numerous social and scientific factors. Thus, error taxonomy and the classification of discrepancy (Table 3) may only help to identify problems and redesign quality process. Pathologists should recognise that they may be unable to provide a reliable evaluation of patient impact if working in isolation from the clinical context; collaboration with or review by relevant clinicians will be needed before plans for remedial action are initiated. In this setting it is important to consider all available information, including information that becomes avail-

Table 3. Description as per duty of care review

Category
1.	No impact on care • No harm: erroneous report not transmitted or received • Near Miss: erroneous report received but ignored or discarded
2.	Minimal harm (no morbidity) • Delay in diagnosis only, <3 months • Unnecessary non-invasive further diagnostic efforts (e.g. Blood sampling, radiograph, computed tomography) • Delay in therapy only, < 3 months • Unnecessary therapy based on diagnostic error without morbidity
3.	Minor harm (minor morbidity)* • Delay in diagnosis only, > 3 months • Unnecessary non-invasive further diagnostic efforts (e.g. biopsy, angiogram) • Delay in therapy only, < 3 months • Delay in therapy with minor morbidity e.g. unnecessary therapy
4.	Moderate harm (Moderate morbidity)** • Moderate morbidity due to delay in diagnosis or therapy • Moderate morbidity due to otherwise unnecessary diagnostic efforts • Moderate morbidity due to otherwise unnecessary therapeutic efforts
5.	Major harm (major morbidity)*** • Loss of limb or an organ or function of an organ system due to unnecessary diagnostic efforts • Severe morbidity due to delayed or unnecessary therapeutic efforts • Death

* Minor morbidity indicates effects and events that can be demonstrated objectively and that do not require admission to hospital or surgical intervention for example, fever, thrombocytopenia, wound erythema, swelling.
** Moderate morbidity indicates effects and events that require admission to hospital or surgical intervention, but do not result in dismemberment or loss of life.
*** Major morbidity indicates dismemberment, loss of an organ or the function of an organ system- an arm/limb, eye/sight, ear/hearing, speech, or the uterus of a woman of reproductive age.

able after the original report was produced. The evaluation should be based on information and material available at the time that the report was issued.

In the context of the evaluation of a doctor's performance, information which became available later is irrelevant, unless this information should have been actively sought before a report was issued; otherwise exercise to evaluate pathologist performance (table 4) is more futile exercise of finding scapegoat.

Table 4. Description with regards to pathologists performance.

Category	
1.	Inadequate dissection, sampling or macroscopic description –where relevant, this should be assessed against guidance such as the college datasets and tissue pathways. It should be remembered that the pathologist issuing the final report may not have dissected, described and sampled the specimen.
2.	Discrepancy in microscopy • A diagnosis which one is surprised to see from any pathologist (e.g. an obvious cancer reported as benign) • A diagnosis which is fairly clearly incorrect, but which one is not surprised to see a small percentage of pathologists suggesting (e.g. a moderately difficult diagnosis, or missing a small clump of malignant cells in an otherwise benign biopsy) • A diagnosis where inter-observer variation is known to be large (e.g. disagreements between two adjacent tumour grades, or any very difficult diagnosis) (Note: In deciding where a specific discrepancy lies in this classification, consideration should be given to the range of responses that might be expected if the case was used in a relevant interpretive external quality assessment scheme.(1) would be surprising diagnosis even from one participant; (2) would be unsurprising from a small minority of participants;(3)would generate diagnoses so varied that the case could not be used for scoring
3.	Discrepancy in clinical correlation – This would represent a failure to answer the clinical question (if clearly expressed on request form), despite that answer being evident from the material available; or a failure to indicate that a specimen is clearly inadequate to answer the clinical question.
4.	Failure to seek a second opinion in an obviously difficult case – This would imply over-confidence
5.	Discrepancy in report – This would include typographical errors and internal inconsistencies or ambiguities in the report which should have been corrected before authorisation.

Conclusions

In trying to define surgical pathology error, most published studies have focused on diagnostic accuracy. However, there is wide spectrum of clinically significant errors occurring in surgical pathology with potential underlying and contributory causes. Examination of the data that the taxonomy uncovers, in root cause analyses, may well reveal that cases of misdiagnosis (the wrong diagnosis for the patient in question) is less often an indictment of the pathologist's diagnostic acumen than problem with implementing and analyzing quality by design. Diagnostic errors may also result from a pathologist making diagnoses on inadequately sampled tissue, either at the gross or microscopic level, when additional material proves diagnostic.

Most often clinicians look to their particular pathology departmental expert as the gold standard, pathologists often view extra-departmental experts of choice as the ultimate measure of diagnostic accuracy. Extra-departmental consultation is limited as an error surveillance tool, given the focus on out-of-the ordinary cases that might be false-negative diagnoses on review. It is important for anatomical pathology department to document and validate error taxonomy in present litigation world.

References

1. Zarbo RJ, Meier FA, Raab SS(2005). Error detection in Anatomic Pathology.Arch Pathol Lab Med. 129:1237-1245.
2. Publications (2006). Concerns about performance in pathology: guidance for healthcare organizations and pathologists. www.rcpath.org/publications

Structural
component of a
quality

Structural
component of a
quality

A quality assurance and improvement plan is merely a small component in maintaining a quality pathology report. Quality in a laboratory depends on a host of structural and personnel factors that are necessary, regardless of the QA& I (quality assurance & improvement) plan. Even better, quality assurance and improvement must be weaved into all the other systems of the laboratory to achieve the absolute best results. Healthcare organizations should recognize that an accurate pathology report requires the collaboration of pathologists, oncology specialists, and other clinicians [1].

The eventual performance outcome of anatomic pathology report is highly dependent not only on the roles of pathologists during the analytic phase but also on the roles clinical practitioners play in pre-analytic and post-analytic phases of the total testing process. It is self-evident that quality gaps still exist due to human factors involved in the process [2]. In the end, pathology report is based on human judgement and is not a computer generated result. Hence, a healthcare organization should concentrate on human structural components of quality in surgical pathology (Healthcare is business; but taking care of a patient is human nature). The following is a discussion of critical elements needed to maintain a quality laboratory.

1. Work force

Flexible, well trained, knowledgeable staffs is key to the success of any organization. This applies to all levels of work within surgical pathology, including pathologists, pathologist's assistant, histology staff, and the secretarial staff. Important aspect of building the staff are qualification, suitability, sufficient redundancy, and the ability to work with others [3]. Of course, individuals must have the appropriate qualification for the job they are doing, but more importantly people must be suited to their duties. Individual with the same qualification may have vastly different strengths and weaknesses and must be placed in positions to take advantage of their strengths, doing the opposite is a sure recipe for failure. In building a workforce, sufficient redundancy in skill is critical to assure continuity or work functions are not affected during an individual's absence. Finally, the staff should work together as a team. The ability to work with others is critical for maintaining a healthy environment and is beneficial to patient safety [4].

2. Continuous education and training

Medical knowledge and treatment is constantly changing. The medical staff must constantly seek out new knowledge and adopt new practices as they become available. These new concepts should be shared and discussed with colleagues, and collectively either adopted or rejected. As individuals are hired they should be trained to the specific peculiarities of their jobs within a particular organization. Individuals should also have regular training in a host of other areas, such as safety and quality improvement, as well as any impending changes in their job duties.

3. The ability to change

Key to the success of most organizations is their ability to respond to changes quickly and effectively. Inherent in these organisations is an ability to adapt and change. While the basis of anatomic pathology practice has not changed significantly over the past half century, changes in the approach to individual diseases are occurring at a much more rapid pace. Breast cancer is a prime example of this evolution. Thirty years ago a pathology report on a breast cancer included a diagnosis and lymph node status. Today a report should include a diagnosis, tumour grade, tumour size, vascular involvement, lymph node status, margin status, and distance to margin if negative, estrogen and progesterone receptor status, Her2/neu immunostain, and possibly a FISH result. Along the way several other factors such as flow cytometry and proliferation markers were at one point thought to be important and were included in pathology reports, but have now been shown to be less significant in determining outcome or treatment and therefore may not need to be included. Although at variable rates, this type of evolution is occurring in many disease processes. A quality anatomic pathology laboratory must remain current with all information to clinicians served by that laboratory.

4. Comprehensive computer system

A comprehensive computer system can greatly enhance the quality of a anatomic pathology laboratory [5]. While all the necessary technology is available, comprehensive computer systems are rare. The ideal system has the ability to pull together all the components of surgical pathology with integrated quality assurance and quality control checks. One may envision a system that allowed physician remote order entry so that the clinical history is mandated and specimens are accounted for as they arrive. A comprehensive system would be tied with an institutional database to confirm the patients identity at accession number and the patient's name and any other identifying information. The system would provide tracking mechanisms through the use of bar code or similar technology, so that all cases, blocks, slides, and reports are accounted for throughout the process. In addition, bar code technology if used to input dictation and transcription so that misidentification errors are reduced. A comprehensive computer system could check and alert if reports have incomplete elements or if cases are not completed within a reasonable time. Such system could then deliver reports electronically to the ordering physician as well as to other venues such as tumour registries. Finally, a comprehensive computer system could generate numerous quality reports in real time and could offer alerts when set parameters are not met.

5. Standardised tasks and language

Quality laboratories have set predetermined standardised procedures that are easily accessible and well known by the staff. A key to quality is the elimination of competing procedures [3]. This is beneficial in reducing confusion over which procedures should be followed, but more importantly it leads to tremendous efficiencies in laboratory operations. Employees must be trained in accepted procedures as they are hired, but also regularly updated as procedures are modified.

Just as important is the standardisation of terms used within the laboratory and in communication with clinicians and physician's office outside of the laboratory, including diagnostic terminology. Diagnostic terminology is constantly being revised and laboratories must have mechanisms to review and update diagnostic criteria and terminology annually. By the token, this needs to be communicated to all who are likely to encounter these terms. To reduce confusion and enhance customer satisfaction, clinicians should be included.

6. Regulatory compliance

Finally, it may be superfluous to say that a laboratory must be in regulatory compliance to operate. Of course this is necessary for licensure, but more importantly, regulatory standards are helpful in guiding laboratories to set up policies and procedures [6]. For the most part regulatory requirements are minimum standards necessary and serve as a foundation for systems and organizational structures to achieve a higher level of quality.

References

1. Nakhleh RE (2006). What is quality in surgical pathology? J Clin pathol 59: 669-672.

2. Crawford JM (2007) Original research in pathology: judgement, or evidence based medicine? Lab Inves 87: 104-114.

3. Spath PL (1999). Reducing errors through work systems improvement. In Spath PL, editor. Error reduction in healthcare. San Francisco: Jassey-Bass, pp 199-234.

4. Grumbach K, Bodenheimer T (2004). Can healthcare teams improve primary care practice? JAMA. 291: 1246-1251.

5. Bates DW (2000). The quality case for information technology in healthcare. BMC Med Informatics Decision Making 2:7-16.

6. Carter DK (2005). Regulatory compliance. In: Nakhleh RE, Fitzgibbons PL, editors. Quality management in anatomic pathology: promoting patients safety through systems improvement and error reduction. Northfield: The college of American Pathologists,pp 9-31.

Join us!

✓ Are you interested in medical publishing?
✓ Are you a skilled scientific writer?
✓ Perhaps wishing to become a dedicated editor of books?

iMedPub is the faster growing medical publishing house and we want to invite you to join. If you have ideas for topics that should be covered by future books, you are welcome to propose new titles in Medicine. Have a look at our blog **The Headhunter** and email us at: info@imedpub.com

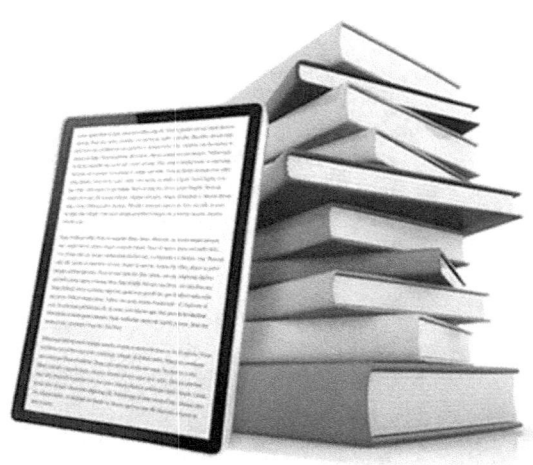

Recent titles by iMedPub:

- *Atlas of Biomarkers for Alzheimer's disease* by Manuel Menendez
- *Point of care testing* by Viroj Wiwanitkit
- *Social Medicine in the 21st Century* by Samuel Barrack
- *Escherichia coli infections* by Viroj Wiwanitkit
- *World Health Report 2012: No Health Without Research* by Samuel Barrack